FLAT BELLY DIET

Lose Weight, Target Belly Fat, and Lower Blood Sugar with This Tested Plan from the Editors of Prevention

Lorelaine Allen

© **Copyright 2021 by Lorelaine Allen- All rights reserved.**

This document is geared towards providing exact and reliable information in regards to the topic and issue covered. The publication is sold with the idea that the publisher is not required to render accounting, officially permitted, or otherwise, qualified services. If advice is necessary, legal or professional, a practiced individual in the profession should be ordered.

- From a Declaration of Principles which was accepted and approved equally by a Committee of the American Bar Association and a Committee of Publishers and Associations.

In no way is it legal to reproduce, duplicate, or transmit any part of this document in either electronic means or in printed format. Recording of this publication is strictly prohibited and any storage of this document is not allowed unless with written permission from the publisher. All rights reserved.

The information provided herein is stated to be truthful and consistent, in that any liability, in terms of inattention or otherwise, by any usage or abuse of any policies, processes, or directions contained within is the solitary and utter responsibility of the recipient reader.

Under no circumstances will any legal responsibility or blame be held against the publisher for any reparation, damages, or monetary loss due to the information herein, either directly or indirectly.

Respective authors own all copyrights not held by the publisher.

The information herein is offered for informational purposes solely, and is universal as so. The presentation of the information is without contract or any type of guarantee assurance.

The trademarks that are used are without any consent, and the publication of the trademark is without permission or backing by the trademark owner. All trademarks and brands within this book are for clarifying purposes only and are the owned by the owners themselves, not affiliated with this document.

Table of contents

INTRODUCTION TO THE BELLY FAT DIET 6

CHAPTER 1: THE DANGERS OF EXCESS BELLY FAT 9

CHAPTER 2: WHAT YOU CAN EXPECT FROM THE BELLY FAT DIET ... 13

CHAPTER 3: EVERYTHING WE THOUGHT WAS WRONG: BLASTING THE MYTHS ABOUT LOSING BELLY FAT 18

CHAPTER 4: HOW TO LOSE YOUR BELLY FAT 26

CHAPTER 5: THE TOP FIVE TOOLS FOR LOSING BELLY FAT FAST AND FOREVER 27

CHAPTER 6: UNDERSTANDING HOW TO BREAK THE CORTISOL CYCLE 37

CHAPTER 7: REVERSING INSULIN RESISTANCE 42

CHAPTER 8: THE SUPPLEMENTS THAT HELP YOU TO LOSE BELLY FAT AND FEEL GREAT WHILE YOU'RE DOING IT 50

CHAPTER 9: EATING MORE TO WEIGH LESS 52

CHAPTER 10: IT'S NOT CHEATING IF IT'S PART OF THE PLAN! 56

CHAPTER 11: THE BELLY FAT DIET FOODS LIST 59

CHAPTER 12: FIVE SUPER-FOODS YOU NEED TO INCLUDE ON YOUR SHOPPING LIST 65

CHAPTER 13: WORKING OUT LESS TO LOOK BETTER THAN EVER ... 69

CHAPTER 14: AN OVERVIEW OF THE WORKOUT PROGRAM 71

CHAPTER 15: AN OVERVIEW OF YOUR MAKEOVER PLAN 75

PUTTING THE BELLY FAT DIET INTO ACTION 77

CHAPTER 16: TWO EXAMPLES FOR YOUR MEAL PLANS 78

CHAPTER 17: TIPS FOR PLANNING YOUR MEALS............................ 81

INTRODUCTION TO THE WORKOUT PLANS 83

THE BELLY FAT DIET SHOPPING GUIDE 91

THE SHOPPING GUIDE 102

INTRODUCTION TO THE BELLY FAT DIET

A flat abdomen has always been the icon of fitness, good health and attractiveness. Every day, there are new diets, workouts and exercise equipment products geared towards losing belly fat and achieving flat, sexy abs.

But losing belly fat isn't just about looking good; it's about being healthy. We now know that excess belly fat is a huge indicator of overall health, especially the risks of heart disease, diabetes and stroke. Losing stored belly fat not only makes you look great and feel better about yourself, it lowers your risk for several diseases and conditions that can greatly affect and even shorten your life. For decades, getting flat abs was viewed as something that required a great deal of hard work and deprivation. Even people who were fairly fit and active complained that they just couldn't shed that tummy pooch or extra five pounds around their middles. Most people attack that stubborn area with thousands of crunches and one new diet after another, and then become frustrated when there are no new results.

The great news is that in the last five years, we've had so much new research into how and why our bodies both store and use belly fat.

Studies done by respected doctors, nutritionists and scientists have revealed that losing stubborn belly fat isn't necessarily about calories, fat grams or crunches. In fact, they've pretty much thrown out all of the things we used to believe about losing belly fat and getting a flat, toned stomach.

Fortunately, that research has also proven that losing belly fat can actually be much faster, easier and more pleasant than anything we used to believe. It doesn't require starvation, hours in the gym or any fancy gadgets or equipment.

The Belly Fat Diet has distilled all of the new research results into one, easy- to-follow plan to help you finally lose that excess fat around your waistline. Best of all, you can do it without being hungry, without spending hours working out or without spending a ton of money on supplements, gym memberships or equipment. You'll eat as much as you want whenever you're hungry, work out as little as twenty minutes per day and feel energized and satisfied.

By following the Belly Fat Diet plan, you'll get dramatic results faster than you ever thought possible and you'll do it without being miserable or sacrificing your health.

We'll provide you with the science behind losing belly fat, as well as a food and shopping guide, recipes, meal plans and a workout program that you'll customize just for you. All you'll need is a commitment to change your body and your health for the better!

Measure Your Risk: A waist measurement of more than half your height in inches indicates serious risk of heart disease, stroke and diabetes. To measure your waist properly, use a measuring tape to measure the circumference of your waist at the belly button. A woman who is 5'4" (64 inches) and has a waist measurement of 32 inches or more is at serious risk of developing these health problems.

Chapter 1: THE DANGERS OF EXCESS BELLY FAT

During a recent television appearance, renowned cardiologist and author Dr. Mehmet Oz caused quite a stir by announcing that your waist measurement is the most important indicator of overall health. During the show, he explained that if your waist measurement is more than half your height (in inches), you are at serious risk for heart disease, stroke and type 2 diabetes. This announcement had many people looking at their measuring tapes not just as a way to measure their fitness, but as a way to measure their future.

Why is excess belly fat so important and what does it have to do with all of these health risks?

Excess Belly Fat Damages Your Liver

Several recent studies on the connection between obesity (particularly excess belly fat) and high levels of liver fat have shown that there is a much higher rate of fatty liver in those with excess belly fat. Fatty liver is a leading indicator of several lipid and metabolic disorders and even liver cancer. In these studies, researchers investigated what makes some obese people develop lipid disorders.

They found that liver fat is strongly associated with increased secretion of very low density lipoproteins (VLDL), which contain the highest amount of triglycerides. High levels of triglycerides carry an increased risk of metabolic abnormalities and increased risk of heart disease and premature death.

Decreasing excess belly fat and blood cholesterol is the recommended treatment for reducing and even reversing fatty liver.

Excess Belly Fat Increases Insulin Resistance and Type 2 diabetes

When we eat, our food, especially carbohydrates, is broken down into glucose so that it can be used to power every cell in our bodies. However, to be used as energy rather than stored as fat, glucose requires the help of insulin.

Insulin is a hormone secreted by the pancreas. Its job is to serve as a key that unlocks your body's cells so that glucose can enter and be used by the cells as energy. Fat cells, particularly abdominal fat cells, lessen the sensitivity to insulin, making it harder for glucose to pass through cell walls. Because the glucose can't enter the cells, it remains in the bloodstream (high blood sugar).

The pancreas responds by producing and releasing more insulin. This cycle repeats itself and grows worse over time. This is what leads to metabolic syndrome and type 2 diabetes.

Excess Belly Fat Greatly Increases the Risk of Heart Disease and Stroke

Because belly fat is so close to the liver (and often accompanied by excess fat directly surrounding the liver), it boosts production of LDL cholesterol (the one we don't want boosted!). This cholesterol eventually becomes a waxy substance known as plaque, which sticks to artery walls and eventually causes swelling, narrowing the arteries. This narrowing increases blood pressure, which seriously taxes the heart. It also increases your chance of blood clots, which can cause stroke.

Excess Belly Fat Increases the Risk of Dementia

Excess belly fat has even been linked to an increased risk of dementia. In fact, excess belly fat increases your risk of developing dementia by as much as 145%! This is a result of the same inflammation in the artery walls, which decreases proper blood flow to the brain.

With all of the serious health risks linked to belly fat, it's easy to see that getting rid of excess belly fat should be a very high priority. Fortunately, while we have lots of "scary" research that shows the risks of belly fat, we also have all of the new research that shows us how to get rid of belly fat quickly, easily and permanently.

Identifying The Two Kinds of Belly Fat

There are actually two kinds of belly fat: subcutaneous fat and visceral fat. Subcutaneous means under the skin. This is the fat you can see and pinch, since it's just below the skin layer.

Visceral fat is the fat that surrounds your vital organs. In the case of abdominal fat, your liver is most commonly affected.

Excess subcutaneous fat around the abdomen is usually accompanied by excess visceral fat around the liver.

The good news: The Belly Fat Diet plan attacks BOTH types of belly fat.

Chapter 2: WHAT YOU CAN EXPECT FROM THE BELLY FAT DIET

You Will Lose Weight, but You Will Also Specifically Lose Belly Fat

Because most diets are designed to help you lose weight by cutting and/or burning calories, they result in weight loss that includes the loss of stored water and lean muscle tissue. If you're able to stick to them for long, you may see a nice new number on the scale, but you still look flabby because you've lost muscle instead of stored fat.

This plan does not rely on simply cutting calories to lose weight. You'll probably take in fewer calories, although some people who have been on low calorie diets will actually start taking in more. The key is that you will be taking in the right calories — from foods that actually help to speed up your metabolism, burn stored fat and utilize your food better to provide energy.

You Will Not be Counting Calories, Carbs or Fat Grams

There are two reasons for this.

This diet does not rely on cutting calories to lose belly fat.

The foods list is designed to provide plenty of nutrition and satisfaction without empty calories, excess carbs or unhealthy fats. As long as you stick to the foods list and follow some simple guidelines, there's no need to track everything you put in your mouth.

You Will Not Be Portioning or Weighing Anything

One of the reasons that most diets fail, even diets that are based on solid science, is that they take too much time to follow correctly. People today are busy; our schedules are already overloaded and our time is already stretched too thinly.

Diets that require you to keep journals, track exchanges and measure, portion and take note of every morsel are a lot like having a second job. No matter how good a diet is, if you don't have time to follow it, it won't work for you.

Again, by sticking to the foods list and following some simple guidelines, you will get plenty of food and plenty of nutrients, without getting too much fat or too many unhealthy carbs. There's nothing to track, nothing to measure.

You Will Not Be Hungry All The Time

One of the keys to losing belly fat is to eat as frequently as possible, even grazing all day long.

Because of this, you won't have to be left feeling hungry or have to suffer through cravings brought on by too little food or a lack of the right nutrients.

It may take your body a week or two to get used to your new way of eating, so you may find yourself feeling hungry frequently. However, when you are hungry, you're supposed to eat! There's no need to deal with a grumbling stomach until the next scheduled meal. Eat!

You Will Not Be Tired and Grumpy

Frequent meals and snacks keep your blood sugar steady. Spikes in blood sugar are quickly followed by crashes in blood sugar. This is the cycle that occurs when you skip meals and then eat a large meal, or get too hungry and grab a snack filled with sugar and simple carbs.

This cycle will leave you feeling fatigued, foggy and irritable. It gets even worse when you limit the good carbs and fats in your diet.

The Belly Fat Diet allows you to eat whenever you want — but you're also eating a diet rich in healthy carbs and fats, so you have a steady supply of energy without all those spikes and crashes.

You Will Probably Lose Weight Faster Than You Expect

It used to be accepted as fact that you should never lose more than two pounds per week. This is because most diets cut calories to lose weight. Losing more than two pounds per week meant that you were reducing your caloric intake to unhealthy levels.

Because the Belly Fat Diet does not rely on this method, but rather helps your body to reset and maximize its fat burning and fat storing systems, you can safely lose more than two pounds per week. The old method of dieting actually caused your body to feed on itself by using its own muscle tissue as a source of protein and energy. With this plan, you'll get plenty of calories, protein and other nutrients. You'll also be resetting your body's fat burning and fat storage systems. This means that the weight you lose will be stored fat, not lean muscle, so it's perfectly safe for you to lose more than two pounds per week.

Some people might lose between five and ten pounds the first week. Do not be concerned that you're losing too much too soon. This is a response to increased metabolism, the shedding of unneeded stored water and targeting stored fat. Weight loss often then levels out in the following weeks to an average of between three and five pounds per week.

Not only will the lean muscle tissue you already have be safe, but you'll also actually be adding more lean muscle on this plan.

"It's Just Water Weight": How many times have you heard that phrase? Fad diets do result in fast initial weight loss and a good deal of that weight is water. However, not all water weight loss is temporary. Excess sodium and processed foods cause your body's tissues to retain excess water. The Belly Fat Diet plan cuts out processed foods, additives and excess sodium, which will stimulate your body to flush out all of that unnecessary fluid. Also, the plan is a permanent lifestyle change, not a quick fix. Hopefully, you won't be going back to an unhealthy diet once you reach your fat loss goals, so you won't be packing that water back on. Therefore, some of the weight you lose in the first week or so will be water, but it won't be coming back.

Chapter 3: EVERYTHING WE THOUGHT WAS WRONG: BLASTING THE MYTHS ABOUT LOSING BELLY FAT

Until very recently, the nutrition and exercise communities had very firm ideas about losing belly fat that went back decades and seemed set in stone. It was considered scientific fact that the only way to lose belly fat was to stick to a very low-calorie, low-fat diet and spend as much time as possible (an hour or more per day was recommended) on strenuous cardio exercise and abdominal workouts.

Excess Belly Fat is Not Your Destiny

This long-held belief about losing belly fat led to a great deal of frustration for dieters. It supported the idea that some people were just genetically predisposed to carry more belly fat, with no hope of redesigning their bodies. Because what we were doing wasn't working, it was assumed that some of us just weren't meant to have flat abs.

The numerous research studies and findings that have come out recently offer a great deal of hope to people who had given up on ever losing that stubborn belly fat. It's much more encouraging to find out that there is a cure for excess belly fat; it just isn't what we thought it was!

Low Calorie Diets Actually Increase Belly Fat

For decades upon decades, it was accepted as simple, scientific fact that the only way to lose fat was to take in fewer calories than you use. We spent years finding our daily caloric requirements (based on sex, age, activity level and height) and figuring out how many calories we needed to cut in order to lose a pound of fat. There were a few things that made this difficult.

First, cutting calories does not specifically address losing belly fat. Second, this mathematical approach to losing weight led many people to cut their caloric intake too low. This brought about a couple of results:

People were unable to maintain such a low-calorie diet, so they found themselves on the yo-yo dieting cycle of losing weight, falling off the diet, gaining back even more weight and starting another low-calorie diet.

Those who were able to stay on their low-calorie diets eventually reached the infamous "weight loss plateau". This is because our metabolisms are designed to conserve energy and store fat (mostly in the abdomen) when they detect a food shortage. If your food intake is too low, your metabolism will virtually shut down to prevent starvation.

We now know that low-calorie diets are almost the opposite of what we need to lose weight, especially to lose belly fat. While you shouldn't take in twice as many calories as you can use in a day, you also shouldn't cut them too low. The balanced answer? Taking in enough (high quality) calories for your body to function efficiently and your metabolism to run at top speed.

Dietary Fat is Not the Enemy

Most of the low-calorie diets we've always been told to follow were also low-fat diets. It was assumed that all fat was bad and that we had to get it out of our diets in order to get it off of our bellies.

The problems are that a) fat is an essential nutrient to our bodies and b) without enough fat, we're unable to stick to our diets and we're back to the yo- yo cycle.

Fat not only enhances the flavor of our food, it also gives us a feeling of satisfaction and fullness, which can curb cravings and prevent overeating. Fat is also used to transport essential vitamins and minerals.

We now know that all fats are not created equal; there are bad fats, good fats and better fats.

Trans-fats, which are found in processed foods and hydrogenated oils, have no place in a healthy diet. Saturated fats, which are found primarily in animal products such as meat and butter, need to be kept to healthy levels. Polyunsaturated fats, such as olive oil, avocado and canola oil are actually good for us, as are the Omega 3 fats found in many fish, nuts and seeds.

The key is not to cut out all fat, but to cut out the bad fats and get plenty of the good ones. The healthy fats not only improve our heart health and brain function; they can also specifically help us to lose belly fat.

Burning a Ton of Calories is Not the Answer

The other long-held belief about losing belly fat was that you had to burn it off by spending hours at the gym or in a class, huffing and puffing your way to a flat belly. Again, this belief came down to math: it was thought that the more calories you burned, the more fat you lost.

Once again, this approach did not specifically target the loss of belly fat. Many people spent hours on the treadmill or in an aerobics class and saw the numbers on the scale drop while the belly fat stayed put. This is what led to the theory that some people are predisposed, by genetics and heredity, to carry more belly fat than others.

This is why we saw a surge in popular diets that claimed to work with your "set point" of weight or BMI or to address certain body types.

Thankfully, we now know that these methods and theories simply failed to address the ways and the reasons that our bodies are designed to store fat or dispose of belly fat. While our genetics and heredity may decide whether we have a long torso or wide shoulders, whether we tend to store fat on our hips or on our thighs, they do not mean that some people can have flat abs and some can't. Anyone can have a slim waist and toned abs. Some of us may have to work harder at it, but we can all achieve it.

All the Crunches in the World Won't Help You Lose Belly Fat

For years, it was accepted as fact that in order to lose belly fat, you had to do specific exercises that targeted the abs. People spent hours doing sit-ups or crunches without seeing results. There's a very simple reason for this: resistance exercise does not burn fat in a specific area. Exercise burns calories and speeds up your metabolism, but your body doesn't burn fat from your abs because you're doing crunches or burn fat from your upper arms because you're doing flies.

Cardio, and to a lesser extent, resistance exercise, burns calories overall. This can help you to lose weight overall and prevent the storage of new fat. However, this is an overall effect, not a targeted effect.

Resistance exercises such as crunches build and tone lean abdominal muscles, but your muscles are located beneath (or behind) the fat layer. This is why you can do loads of crunches and still have a fat tummy. The muscles are there, you just can't see them. In order for those crunches to result in a flat, toned tummy, you have to get rid of the fat that's hiding those muscles.

Before you get discouraged about all those wasted crunches, understand that the exercise you've been doing and the exercise you're about to do will soon pay off. If you've been working out regularly, those muscles are under there, you just need to reveal them. The Belly Fat Diet is going to help you do that, and much more quickly and easily than you're probably thinking.

Our bodies have very specific systems, checks and balances for utilizing, storing and disposing of stored fat. By using what we have learned about these processes and working with them, we can finally lose the excess belly fat that has stubbornly refused to budge.

By making some simple and even very pleasant (how does snacking all day and getting a good night's rest sound?) diet and lifestyle changes, we can finally transform our bodies into lean, toned, fat-burning machines without having to live the life of an athlete or eating the diet of a bird.

In the next section, we'll explain these fat burning and fat storing processes and how you can use them to finally get the body you've always wanted.

Chapter 4: How to Lose Your Belly Fat

- *The Top Five Tools for Losing Belly Fat Fast and Forever*
- *Understanding How to Break the Cortisol Cycle*
- *Reversing Insulin Resistance*
- *The Supplements That Help You Lose Belly Fat and Feel Great Doing It*
- *Eating More to Weigh Less*
- *It's Not Cheating If It's Part of The Plan!*
- *The Belly Fat Diet Foods List*
- *Five Super-Foods You Need to Include on Your Shopping List*
- *Working Out Less to Look Better Than Ever*
- *An Overview of Your Makeover Plan*

Chapter 5: THE TOP FIVE TOOLS FOR LOSING BELLY FAT FAST AND FOREVER

The Belly Fat Diet takes all of the current research and all of the new findings about losing belly fat and incorporates them into one, effective and easy-to- follow plan.

The plan addresses:

- How cortisol controls the storage and disposal of belly fat and how you can break the cortisol cycle.
- How and why the hormones leptin and ghrelin can work for or against belly fat loss.
- The role insulin plays in both storing excess belly fat and regulating cravings and energy levels.
- The connection between stress and excess belly fat and how to break it. The role of vitamin C and Omega 3 fats in losing belly fat.
- How to boost your metabolism to burn more fat all day long.
- The most effective exercise method for losing weight and belly fat.

Tool # 1: Breaking the Cortisol Cycle

There's been so much information in the media and in diet books about the role that cortisol plays in the storage and disposal, or burning, of belly fat. If you haven't read the research or done much investigating on your own, you may not understand what cortisol is, what it does and how to break the cortisol cycle.

Cortisol is one of the stress hormones naturally produced and secreted in the body. Cortisol's specific job is to react to stress signals by storing fat in the abdominal area. The reason this system exists is because, in ages past, stress often indicated a chance of famine in the near future. Back when people moved from place to place to find food and were often considered food themselves by other predators, stress was a signal that we were on the run and food was going to be in short supply.

Very few of us are in danger of famine from the stress we're under today, but the body's system for storing fat in times of stress remains in place. To our bodies, stress is stress, whether it's from a shortage of food, a lion who thinks we look like dinner, or a boss who wants us to work long hours.

This is where the cortisol cycle comes in. We're more stressed today than people have ever been before. We have financial problems, busy schedules, demanding jobs and families to take care of in between. That stress triggers the release of cortisol into our bloodstreams, which causes our bodies to direct fat to the abdomen to be used in case of famine. The problem is, there is no famine. We continue to eat more than enough food, so that fat is never used as an energy source.

We'll tell you more in depth what you need to know about cortisol in the next few pages, but the Belly Fat Diet will break the cortisol cycle and reset your system so that your body uses dietary fat properly but also gets rid of the fat it already has stored up on your abdomen.

Tool #2: Reversing Insulin Resistance

Your hormones are at it again! Like cortisol, insulin is a hormone produced by your body, although it is not a stress hormone. The role of insulin is to regulate the amount of sugar in your bloodstream and to allow glucose (created from the foods you eat) to be used by cells as energy.

You may have heard about insulin resistance, which is a situation where your body's cells become resistant to insulin and glucose cannot pass through the cell membrane to be used as energy. When this occurs, two things happen:

1... your blood sugar levels spike and drop repeatedly, causing a fatigue/energy boost/fatigue cycle.

2... all of that unused glucose is stored as fat, mainly around your belly.

Like the situation with stress, cortisol and belly fat, insulin resistance is cyclical. The cycle goes something like this:

Excess belly fat makes your body resistant to insulin. Insulin resistance causes your body to store more belly fat. Rinse and repeat.

This cycle is what can eventually lead to type 2 diabetes, which is why excess belly fat is a leading indicator of developing the disease. Fortunately, this cycle is reversible. In fact, even if you already have type 2 diabetes, losing belly fat and making the dietary changes prescribed in the Belly Fat Diet can greatly improve and even reverse the disease!

Tool #3: Vitamin C

Vitamin C has always been known as the wonder vitamin when it comes to preventing and relieving colds and other infections.

However, the importance of vitamin C goes far beyond fighting infection and boosting immunity.

Vitamin C is also one of the key players in losing belly fat. It does this in two ways:

First, vitamin C is a necessary for the production of L-carnitine, a chemical used to transport stored fat, particularly abdominal fat, to where it can be burned as energy.

Second, vitamin C reduces the effects of stress on the body, which helps to break the cortisol cycle, so that your body is stimulated to both burn stored belly fat and to stop storing new belly fat.

Vitamin C is a soluble vitamin, which means that our bodies don't store it up in great quantities. We use a great deal of it for cell renewal and cell production and most of the rest of it is spent fighting off infection. Unfortunately, stress also uses up a great deal of vitamin C.

This means we have yet another cycle that gets in the way of losing that belly fat. We're stressed, so we have excess cortisol released into our bloodstreams, causing our bodies to store belly fat. That stress we're under also uses up all of our extra vitamin C, so there isn't enough L-carnitine to move that belly fat to where it can be repurposed as energy.

On the Belly Fat Diet plan, you'll be getting a great deal of vitamin C from your diet, which will be full of vitamin C-dense foods. But you'll also be taking a vitamin C supplement twice per day to give your body the extra C it needs to burn the belly fat you already have. This vitamin C supplementation is essential to turbo-charging the belly fat loss in the first few weeks. As an added bonus, you'll be boosting your immune system through both the vitamin C and your antioxidant-rich diet.

Tool #4: Getting Leptin and Ghrelin on Your Side

You've met cortisol; now let us introduce you to leptin and ghrelin. Both are hormones that greatly influence your weight by controlling your appetite. Leptin is secreted in fat tissue and sends a signal to your brain that lets it know you're full. Ghrelin is secreted in the intestinal tract and sends signals indicating that you're hungry.

Leptin and ghrelin aren't stress hormones, but they do have something in common with cortisol: they are impacted by your sleep habits. Several recent research studies have shown that people who get less than seven hours of sleep per night have elevated ghrelin levels and decreased leptin levels.

One of the interesting findings in these studies is that one night of missed or interrupted sleep is enough to see this change in leptin and ghrelin levels.

It's far more pronounced when insufficient sleep is a regular pattern, but one all-night study session or party into the wee hours is enough to interfere with the work of these two hormones.

What this means for you is that getting adequate (7-8 hours minimum) sleep, preferably at the same time each night, is essential to keeping leptin and ghrelin on your side. It won't take long to get them regulated, so that you'll soon be overeating less and seeing fewer hunger pangs. This translates to faster belly fat loss without having to do anything other than sleep!

Fish Oil Helps You Lose Belly Fat: The DHA and EPA in Omega-3 fats have been shown to reduce symptoms of depression and signs of stress, which can help you to avoid emotional eating. Studies have also shown that people who eat plenty of oily fish and other Omega-3 rich foods lose more fat per week than dieters who don't; on average one pound more. The Belly Fat Diet is filled with Omega-3 fats from fish, shellfish, avocadoes, olive oil, nuts and seeds. You'll also be taking a fish oil supplement each day. It'll be good for your heart, your mood and your waistline.

Tool #5: Interval Training

If you've read or heard about interval training, you may have thought it was just for athletes and those who are already pretty fit. The truth is, anyone can utilize interval training to maximize the effects of their workouts in a minimum of time. Interval training is simply alternating periods of moderate work with shorter bursts of more intense work. You can apply it to virtually any form of exercise and you can start right where you are, even if you haven't done a bit of exercise in years. The wonderful thing is that your body reacts to the level of exertion you require for your workouts, so beginners can benefit just as much as athletes.

Interval training has been proven to be far more effective than a static (steady paced) workout. In fact, twenty minutes of interval training boosts your metabolism longer than an hour of static exercise!

Interval training works because your body adjusts itself very quickly to your workouts. As you become stronger, your metabolism works less to achieve the same number of reps or the same mileage walked. What this usually means is that people discover they have to work out longer to get the same results.

With interval training, you are constantly keeping your body guessing, so your metabolism is never given a chance to adjust and slow down.

This metabolism boost means that you'll burn more calories throughout the day, no matter what you're doing. This allows you to lose fat faster without cutting calories. Another benefit to interval training is that you don't have to spend hours working out. You can spend just twenty or thirty minutes a day on interval training. As you progress, you won't add more time to your workouts, you'll simply adjust the moderate periods to be shorter or more intense and adjust the intense periods to be longer or more difficult, still keeping your total workout time down to twenty or thirty minutes.

There's one more benefit to interval training, too. Interval training builds lean muscle faster than steady training. Lean muscle not only burns more calories than fat tissue, but it also improves the efficiency with which glucose is absorbed and burned by muscles. (Remember that glucose absorption has everything to do with reducing your risk of diabetes and losing stored belly fat.)

Conclusion

These five tools represent the best that all of the new research into fat loss and belly fat have to offer.

We've taken all of them and put them into one easy-to- follow plan that will help you burn that belly fat faster than you thought possible, all while helping you to feel satisfied and energetic.

With these tools, losing that stubborn belly fat is not only possible, it's enjoyable.

Chapter 6: UNDERSTANDING HOW TO BREAK THE CORTISOL CYCLE

We've explained what cortisol is and what it does in the previous chapter. Now you need to know why cortisol is released into the bloodstream and how the Belly Fat Diet will help you to break the cortisol cycle and finally get rid of your excess belly fat quickly, painlessly and permanently.

As you read earlier, cortisol is a stress hormone. When your body perceives stress, it signals the release of cortisol into the bloodstream. That cortisol release stimulates the storage of fat around your belly, specifically on a part of your abdomen known as the omentum. The omentum is a layer of deep tissue that stretches across your abdomen behind the navel. This is why the measurement of your waist at the belly button is such an important indicator of your risk for the diseases and conditions attributed to excess belly fat.

It Doesn't Take A Lot of Stress to Stimulate Cortisol Release

This is an important fact to keep in mind. A recent study on cortisol and belly fat revealed that even the stress of counting calories increased cortisol levels in the bloodstream.

While major stressors such as unemployment, the death of a loved one or divorce stimulate the release of more cortisol, the minor stressors of daily life add up to a good deal of cortisol in your bloodstream — enough to keep that belly fat growing.

The Other Factors that Stimulate Cortisol Release

The stress of everyday life and the major stressors we all encounter from time to time are not the only things that will increase cortisol production and release. Cortisol release will also be stimulated by insufficient or irregular sleep and hunger, and skipping meals.

The Belly Fat Diet addresses these factors in order to help you break the cortisol cycle. In order to reduce the amount of cortisol coursing through your system, you will:

Forget about counting calories, measuring grams, weighing portions or writing down everything you eat. As we've said before, these tactics that have been so popular on other diets actually make the diets hard to stick with for any length of time. Now you know they also stress you out enough to stimulate cortisol production and keep you from losing that belly fat.

Get a minimum of seven hours sleep every night, on a regular schedule. We've already explained that getting sufficient and regular sleep is essential to keeping the hormones leptin and ghrelin working for you, not against you.

It's also one of the most important things you can do to break the cortisol cycle. Several research studies have been released in the last few years that investigated the link between insufficient sleep, cortisol levels and body fat ratios. All of these studies reported that people who get at least seven hours of sleep each night at fairly regular times (going to bed within the same one to two hours each night) are more likely to weight less, have smaller body fat ratios and slimmer waistlines than those who regularly sleep less than seven hours. Remember that old line about "losing weight while you sleep"? It was almost true!

Eat as often as possible, with no more than two hours between meals and snacks. This one may be music to a dieter's ears, but it's based on solid, scientific research.

Going more than two or three hours without eating:

- Causes a sharp drop in blood sugar, creating cravings for unhealthy carbs and sugars.
- Slows the metabolism.

- Increases cortisol levels in the blood.
- Causes fatigue and mental fogginess that has us reaching for coffee, sodas and candy bars.
-

On the Belly Fat Diet eating plan, you can eat anything on the foods list as often as possible without overeating or stuffing yourself. You'll also need to be sure to eat as soon after waking as you possibly can. This kick-starts your metabolism, keeps your blood sugar at a healthy level and keeps cortisol from overreacting to eight hours without food.

There's one other thing you can do to positively impact cortisol function: have at least fifteen minutes a day that is devoted to unwinding, loosening up, laughing and de-stressing by any means that works for you. Use a fifteen minute coffee break to get outdoors or listen to some soothing music with the office lights turned down. Play with your kids or your dog when you get home to help you detox from the little (or not so little) stresses of your day. Incorporate some yoga or yoga breathing into your workout plan. Everyone has their favorite way to let go of stress; find several of yours and use them throughout the week. If you have fifteen minutes for a phone call, surfing the web or leafing through a magazine, you have fifteen minutes to take care of yourself.

Fortunately, it doesn't take long to get your cortisol levels in line. Within a couple of weeks of starting the Belly Fat Diet, you'll have cortisol working to help you shed that belly fat.

Chapter 7: REVERSING INSULIN RESISTANCE

As we explained previously, insulin resistance is a common result of excess belly fat. It may be a bit of a chicken-or-egg type situation as well. Insulin resistance causes excess belly fat to be stored because glucose is not being used as energy. At the same time, excess belly fat and the eating patterns that cause it can also create insulin resistance.

As with correcting the cortisol cycle, avoiding, reducing and reversing insulin resistance is achieved through dietary changes, reducing belly fat and moderate exercise. Many studies have concluded that even if you already have type 2 diabetes, you can greatly improve or even reverse it through making these lifestyle and health changes.

Fighting Insulin Resistance through Healthy Eating

The Belly Fat Diet eating plan works on correcting or preventing insulin resistance in four ways:

- Eliminating almost all processed foods, which are filled with sugar and refined flour.
- Reducing overall sugar intake.

- Increasing protein and plant fiber intake to slow absorption of carbs. Frequent meals and snacks to keep blood sugar steady.

- Processed Foods are Not Your Friends

There are almost no processed foods allowed on the eating plan. This means no fast food, no convenience foods, no ready-made baked goods and so on. Processed foods such as these are filled with refined flours and other starches that are broken down very quickly and create a sharp increase in blood glucose levels. Your body responds with an equally sharp increase in insulin. Twenty minutes to an hour later, your blood sugar drops just as rapidly and you reach for another quick boost, usually more carbs and sugar. This cycle is credited as being one of the main causes of insulin resistance.

Carbohydrates from grains are limited on the eating plan because they're one of the easiest to overeat and among the fastest to be turned into sugar by your body's digestive system. Whole grain oatmeal and multi-grain cereals, whole grain bread and a few other high-fiber grains are allowed on the diet in limited quantities, but most of your fiber will come from plant foods, which are absorbed much more slowly.

The Eating Plan is Very Low in Added Sugar

Too much sugar in your diet presents the same problems as too much refined flour and processed food: it's absorbed very quickly into the bloodstream and wreaks havoc on your blood sugar and your insulin sensitivity.

Added sugars are allowed on the eating plan, but in much smaller quantities than many people usually eat. If at all possible, you should limit it to sweetening your coffee or tea (if you need it) and the amounts that naturally occur in allowed foods such as flavored Greek yogurts, frozen fruit bars and some of the homemade sweet treats we've included in the Belly Fat Diet Cookbook.

At first, you may balk at having to ration your sweets, but after a couple of weeks, your sugar cravings will be much more easily satisfied by healthier sweets such as fresh fruit, which you can eat freely on the diet.

High Protein and Fiber Intake Keeps Blood Sugar Steady

One of the other efficient ways to end the spike and drop cycle in blood sugar levels is to slow the absorption of carbs and sugars.

You may have heard or read about the glycemic index, which measures foods based on how quickly they are absorbed into the bloodstream as glucose. Examples of high-glycemic foods would be table sugar, cake, cookies and candy. Healthier foods can also have a relatively high glycemic index. Bananas rate high on the index, as do dried fruits. On the other hand, meats, eggs, cheese and vegetables such as spinach rank very low because they are converted to glucose much more slowly.

In addition to the glycemic index, there is something called the glycemic load, which is the total glycemic index of a meal or combination of foods. Some foods, when combined, create a lower glycemic load. For instance, if you have a banana by itself, its glycemic index is high, but if you have a banana with three scrambled eggs the total glycemic load is quite low.

This is because protein and fiber, when eaten with a carb food such as bread or fruit, slow the absorption of those carbs into the bloodstream. This results in a much slower rise in blood sugar after a meal, which is easily dealt with by insulin release. It also gets rid of that pesky carb crash.

On the Belly Fat Diet eating plan, you're encouraged to include a protein or high-fiber food in every meal and snack. For instance, if you feel like having an orange, we encourage you to have a mozzarella stick or boiled egg, too. This will not only lower the glycemic load of that orange, it will also keep you feeling more satisfied than if you eat the orange alone.

Frequent Meals Increase Insulin Sensitivity

As mentioned previously, frequent meals help you to reduce or avoid insulin resistance because you eliminate the blood sugar spikes and drops that come with skipping meals. You'll also be less likely to reach for forbidden snacks such as colas or candy bars to fight sluggishness. Even further, it's been shown that eating smaller, more frequent meals helps prevent overeating. Even with healthy foods, it's possible to eat too much if you let yourself get too hungry.

Improving Insulin Sensitivity through Exercise

One of the first things doctors advise patients with type 2 diabetes, metabolic syndrome or insulin resistance is to get moving. Physicians strongly urge patients who either have these issues or are at risk for them to get at least some cardiovascular (or aerobic) and resistance (or strength training) exercise each week. This is also a huge component of the Belly Fat Diet.

The ways that exercise improves insulin sensitivity can get a little complicated and explaining them can get a little too technical, so we'll break it down into a somewhat oversimplified, two-step process.

Let's start with the two types of effects that exercise has on insulin sensitivity. They're known as the acute (or immediate and temporary) effect and the training (long term) effect. Studies have shown conclusively that even a single bout of moderate exercise improves insulin sensitivity for a short period of time; anywhere from twelve hours to two days. This is the acute effect. These same studies show that regular, moderate exercise soon results in a round-the-clock improvement in insulin sensitivity. This is known as the training effect.

Moderate cardiovascular exercise, such as twenty to thirty minutes of walking, biking, swimming or dancing, is enough for your body reap the benefits of increased insulin sensitivity.

The same is true of resistance training. However, resistance training offers some extra benefits.

When you train your muscles, they use glycogen (the form of glucose that is stored in muscle and used as energy) to both provide energy and rebuild muscle tissue. They also continue to "request" glucose for up to 24 hours after the workout. This means that there's less glucose roaming around in your bloodstream and less insulin needed to deal with it. That is the acute effect of resistance training.

However, there are actually two types of training effects created by resistance or strength training. First, regular strength training produces the training effect that we've already discussed. Second, the more lean muscle you have, the more efficiently your body uses glucose and insulin overall. Fat tissue doesn't need glucose, it stores it. Muscle tissue uses glucose for energy. The more lean muscle you have, the more glucose you need and the less glucose you have being added to fat stores, especially around your tummy.

We'll provide more detail and several workout plans in the exercise section, but the Belly Fat Diet includes twenty to thirty minutes of cardio exercise at least three times per week and twenty to thirty minutes of resistance training at least three times per week. That's enough to get your insulin sensitivity back to maximum performance and help you to Belly Fat Diet and build a leaner, stronger body.

Many people report noticing a change in their energy levels, mood, cravings and hunger (signs of improved insulin sensitivity) almost immediately, but expect it to take a couple of weeks for you to see a real difference.

Note: You should talk to your doctor before starting any diet or exercise program, but if you've been diagnosed with type 2 diabetes, it is particularly essential that you let your doctor know your plans (for both diet and exercise) before you get started.

Chapter 8: THE SUPPLEMENTS THAT HELP YOU TO LOSE BELLY FAT AND FEEL GREAT WHILE YOU'RE DOING IT

While the Belly Fat Diet eating plan is filled with foods that are packed with vitamins, minerals, antioxidants and other essential micronutrients, you'll also be taking a few select supplements that will further nourish your body and help you to lose that belly fat.

It's best to get your doctor's okay before starting on a supplement program, so do discuss the list with your doctor before you begin. In some cases, current health issues and regular medications may require some adjustment.

The Daily Supplement Plan

Each morning and evening (or late afternoon), you'll be taking:

- 1000mg vitamin C (chewable tablets are fine) 1000mg of a high-quality fish oil supplement
- 1 B-Vitamin Complex (ask your doctor for recommended dosage)

We've already discussed vitamin C at length and its importance in reducing cortisol and producing L-Carnitine to transport stored fat. Because vitamin C is a soluble vitamin, our bodies don't store much; any excess will be disposed of as waste, so there's no need to worry about taking too much unless if you get into mega-dosing (amounts ranging from 5,000 to 10,000 daily).

The fish oil supplement is an added dose of healthy Omega-3 fats to supplement those you're getting through your diet. Be sure to read the labels and even ask for help at the health food store or pharmacy where you purchase it. You want a supplement that contains both DHA and EPA. If you really don't care for fish and seafood, you may want to ask your doctor about increasing the amount of fish oil you take daily, as you'll be getting less of it through your diet. The B-complex of vitamins are also soluble vitamins. Since our bodies don't store them in any real quantity, most of our supply has to come through our daily diet. The fruits and vegetables you'll be eating will provide a healthy supply, but taking a supplement insures that your immune system and energy levels are getting all they need.

Chapter 9: EATING MORE TO WEIGH LESS

The Belly Fat Diet eating plan allows you to eat as much of the allowed foods as you want, as often as possible. This will keep hunger and cravings at bay, keep your energy high, your blood sugar steady and just make you a whole lot happier and more willing to stick with the plan.

However, there are some guidelines to follow.

Eating as Much as You Want Does Not Mean Loading Up Your Plate

Unless you're piling raw veggies on your plate, you need to use some common sense about how much to eat at once.

Part of reshaping the way you eat is helping your body to be happy with "just enough" food. This means that if you're having chicken breast, a salad and a baked sweet potato for dinner, you should eat slowly and finish everything before deciding you want more. If you are still hungry, by all means, have another breast or some more veggies. However, your goal should be to eat just until satisfied, not until stuffed. Overstuffing your digestive system is counterproductive to your goals and makes you feel sluggish and uncomfortable.

Did you know? It really does take about 20 minutes for your body to register the food you're eating. For meals, make sure you take at least twenty minutes to eat. Then decide if you're still hungry.

Learn to Read Your Hunger

As your body adjusts to a healthier diet and your hormones begin to cooperate with you, you'll experience fewer cravings, especially for sweets. This usually takes about two weeks. However, you'll have those times when you're hungry, especially in the first few weeks. It's perfectly okay to eat, but for those times when you're standing in front of the fridge, unsure of what it is you want, try satisfying yourself with these foods in this order:

- Try some water — thirst often masks itself as hunger.
- If you're still hungry or just know you crave actual chewing, try a vegetable.
- If you're still hungry, try a fruit.
- If you're still hungry, go for a protein.

(You get grains in such limited quantities; don't waste them on a random nosh.)

Why is this order important? For those times when you know you're not truly hungry but are just bored or need something to crunch or chew, trying these foods in this order will keep you from reaching for the higher calorie, higher fat and higher carbs foods first and eating more than you need to satisfy an urge that isn't really hunger-based.

This is not the same situation as planned snacks and meals. This is for eating out of boredom, stress or nervousness, or what is commonly called emotional eating.

Your Three Limitations: Beef, Sweet Treats and Grains

There are only three food categories that carry some limitations. They are beef, grains and sweet treats.

Beef is limited because it typically contains a good deal of unhealthy fats, is expensive to buy in healthier, grass-fed varieties and is usually eaten in fairly large portions. You're limited to one serving per week of steak or roast; the leaner cut the better, trimmed of visible fat. If you don't eat beef, that's all the better. If you truly love it and doing without it every day is going to be a challenge, reward yourself with your favorite steak once a week.

Most grains are limited because they are easy to overeat, quickly converted to sugar or glucose and many of them fail to fill you up for very long. You're limited to two servings per day of the grains on the allowed foods list.

Sweet treats are allowed on the eating plan, but they're limited to one per day and only the sweet treats that are on the allowed foods list. These are few, but tasty. They include frozen fruit pops, nonfat pudding, sorbet and dark chocolate. Use moderation is your servings of these foods and try to really enjoy them. Eat them at a time when you can focus on how good they taste, rather than eating them mindlessly or in a rush.

Chapter 10: IT'S NOT CHEATING IF IT'S PART OF THE PLAN!

Now that you've heard about the few limitations and rules of the eating plan, it's time to let you in on one guideline that will probably be quite welcome. You're supposed to cheat.

Once a week, you are allowed to have one thing that you've been craving, missing, waiting for and doing without. If your true love is pizza, have it. If you've been going through milkshake withdrawal, get one.

Of course, you need to use a bit of sense here. You're not supposed to have a whole pizza, but a slice or two. If you can make it a thin crust veggie pizza, that would be awesome, but if Hawaiian with extra cheese is the only thing that makes you happy, have it. Any kind, with any of the enemies you feel like loading on top of it — but just have one or two slices.

If you've been waiting all week for Fettuccine Alfredo, then you deserve to really enjoy it … a sensible portion of it.

If you've been dying for a Snickers, some dinner rolls and some chips, we're afraid you're going to have to pick one. The others can be your cheat for next week.

Some Guidelines to Help You Cheat the Right Way

Aside from the One Cheat Once Per Week rule and the caution about portions, there are a few tips and guidelines that can help you cheat the right way.

If you're longing for a few different foods, try to choose the one that is either the healthiest or highest in protein.

If one coveted food has sugar and the other doesn't, opt for the one without sugar. It'll affect insulin and blood sugar less.

Try to choose foods you really love, rather than wasting your weekly cheat on something that just shows up. In other words, don't give in to an unplanned slice of mediocre cake at an office party when you've been looking forward to having gourmet ice cream on Saturday.

Why You're Supposed to Cheat

The answer to this may seem obvious, but it bears explaining anyway. There are actually a few reasons why it's a good idea to plan a controlled, weekly cheat.

Knowing you're going to have that gourmet ice cream Saturday makes it easier to do without your usual nightly bowl.

Going without your favorite foods indefinitely leads to frustration, resentment and out-of-control cheating. Limiting yourself to your daily sweet and a weekly cheat takes some getting used to at first, but it's much easier than going without altogether.

This means you have a much better chance of sticking to the plan until you've reached your goals….and being happier while you do.

Eventually, you'll reach your fat loss goals and be ready to move on to a more lenient diet. However, you need to have healthy habits in place when you do or you'll be right back where you started before too long. Putting off indulgences and using some sense when indulging are habits that have to be learned, but they'll serve you well later on.

Truthfully, life is hard enough. No bread lover should have to live without yeast rolls forever. You're working hard at changing your health and your body. You deserve a weekly cheat and if done right, it won't undo any of that hard work.

Chapter 11: THE BELLY FAT DIET FOODS LIST

In the included Belly Fat Diet Shopping Guide, you'll find a much more detailed list of the foods you're allowed to eat on the Belly Fat Diet eating plan. You may want to make several copies and circle items as you plan your menus and your grocery shopping.

Here, we'll give you an overview of what you'll be eating.

Meat and Poultry

You're free to eat chicken breast or ground chicken breast, turkey breast or ground turkey breast and eggs as often as you like. If you want to make sandwiches or salads with these meats, please use leftover home cooked poultry rather than packaged or deli counter meats. Those contain far too much sodium and too many nitrates and preservatives.

You're allowed lean cuts of beef steak or beef roast once a week.

Fish and Seafood

You can have as much fish and seafood as you like, as long as it isn't breaded, fried or covered in a cream sauce. It should be steamed, broiled, baked, boiled or sautéed in a bit of olive or canola oil.

Try to focus on oily, cold water fish, as they're the richest in Omega-3 fats. On the foods list, we've listed those varieties for you. However, you're free to eat any variety you like.

Dairy Products

Dairy products are limited to skim or reduced fat milk, low-fat or nonfat mozzarella and cottage cheese and Greek yogurt. (Greek yogurt has twice the protein of regular yogurt so it has more staying power and balances out the sugar.)

Try to limit the milk to using for coffee, cereal and cooking, rather than using it as a beverage. Milk is actually a food, not a drink. This will keep your intake down to a healthy level. However, if a cold glass of milk is a real treat for you, go ahead and have it, just keep it down to one glass a day.

Butter and butter substitutes are off-limits, as are other cheeses.

Fruits and Vegetables

You can have any fruit you like, as often as you like. Fresh is best, but frozen fruits (without syrup or added sugar) are fine for out-of-season fruits or for adding to smoothies and other treats.

When using fruit as a snack, try to couple it with a protein to lessen the effect on your blood sugar. For example, if you're in the mood for some grapes, have them with a stick of mozzarella or a boiled egg.

All vegetables are allowed on the plan, with the exception of white potatoes and corn. Both are high in starch, which means they're quickly converted to sugar.

Veggies are best eaten raw, but steaming, roasting, baking, sautéing and stir- frying are perfectly fine. As with fruits, fresh veggies are best but frozen vegetables without butter sauce or cheese sauce added are perfectly acceptable.

Canned fruits and veggies are off limits, as they usually contain fewer vitamins and minerals, less fiber and a good deal of sugar and additives.

Grains

Grains are a good source of fiber, but most of them are converted to sugar quite quickly. They're also one of the easiest foods to overeat. For this reason, grains are limited to two servings per day and you may choose from whole-wheat, whole grain breads and cereals, brown rice, quinoa, barley and whole grain oats.

When you're choosing your grains, it's a good idea to opt for the most filling choice. A slice of whole grain toast won't stick with you for long, but a bowl of mixed-grain hot cereal will.

Nuts, Seeds and Oils

Nuts and seeds can be an excellent source of healthy fats and fiber, as long as you eat the right ones. Walnuts and almonds are your best choice and should be eaten either raw or roasted without salt or sugar. You may also have almond butter or sesame butter that has no trans-fats or sugar added. Avocadoes, olive oil and canola oil are also allowed, as well as pumpkin, sesame and poppy seeds.

Condiments and Sweet Treats

Refer to the included Belly Fat Diet Shopping Guide for a more detailed list, but condiments that are not packed with sugars and unhealthy fats are allowed. Ketchup, mayonnaise and Miracle Whip are off limits.

You've already heard about the sweet treats that you can choose from daily,

but to repeat, they include frozen fruit pops with no added sugar, sorbets without added sugar, nonfat pudding (the sugared variety, rather than artificially sweetened — no artificial sweeteners are allowed on the plan) and dark chocolate. Limit yourself to one pop, one pudding cup, one scoop of sorbet and one piece of chocolate the size of a dental floss box.

Beverages

Beverages are limited to water, coffee, green tea and black tea. You can sweeten your coffee and tea if you must, but limit the sugar in the rest of your diet to accommodate. Black coffee is better than coffee with milk, but milk is allowed while artificial and flavored creamers are not.

You need to drink a minimum of 64 ounces of plain water per day, more if you spend a good deal of time outdoors.

Juices are not on the diet because they contain little or no fiber, don't fill you up like the whole fruit will and are easy to overdo. The same is true of flavored waters. Sodas are strictly off limits. Save them for your cheat day if you're really attached to your colas.

Other allowed foods include unsweetened protein powder, honey, agave nectar (as a sugar substitute) all herbs and seasonings and a few other items that will make it easier for you to plan delicious and nutritious meals. The grocery list in the Belly Fat Diet Shopping Guide will give you a more complete rundown of what's allowed.

Chapter 12: FIVE SUPER-FOODS YOU NEED TO INCLUDE ON YOUR SHOPPING LIST

All of the foods included on the Belly Fat Diet are extremely healthy and taste great to boot. However, there are some real superstars in the food world: foods that have become known as "super-foods" in the nutritional community.

There are a number of foods that have been given their fifteen minutes of well-deserved fame recently. These include berries, soybeans and soy products, acai and many others. They're all nutritional winners, but no single food will give you everything you need. A variety of these extremely valuable foods is what you need to see a drastic change in how you look and feel.

We've highlighted five stars that are easily found in your local store, very affordable and generally well-liked by most people. Keep these on your running grocery list and eat at least one of them each day to give your immune system an extra boost.

Berries

Berries are loaded with vitamin C and several of the B-vitamins. They're also packed with phytonutrients and antioxidants.

The darker the color, the better they are for you. Cranberries, black raspberries, blueberries and blackberries are all excellent choices.

Salmon

Salmon is one of the best fish choices for getting Omega-3 fatty acids. If salmon is too rich for either your taste buds or your budget, sardines, mackerel, tuna, cod and other cold water fish are equally good, but more affordable choices.

Nuts

Nuts have gotten a bad rap, mostly because people don't understand the difference between healthy fats and unhealthy ones, but also because many of us tend to indulge in varieties that aren't that great for you, such as macadamias and cashews. Nuts provide protein, heart-healthy fats, a ton of insoluble fiber and a bonus dose of antioxidants. Walnuts and almonds are your healthier choices and you should eat them in as natural a state as possible. Raw is best, roasted okay, too, as long as you skip the salted or honey-roasted types.

Kiwi

Kiwi is a nutritional jackpot, but also one of the most affordable super-foods around.

Sometimes available for as little a dime each, these tasty gems are a nutritional bargain. They're packed with vitamin C and fiber, and have few calories.

Sweet Potatoes

These delicious and nutritious vegetables are one of the many orange veggies that make the various super-foods lists. They're very cheap, are packed with antioxidants, have a good amount of protein and are high in fiber. They also contain a healthy dose of Vitamin C. One of the nice things about sweet potatoes is that they satisfy the sweet tooth, too. Roast or bake them and flavor with a bit of olive oil, salt and pepper and you'll never miss the butter or that less-healthy white baked potato you used to eat.

There are many other foods we could include on this list, but adding just these five to your daily diet every week will have a terrific impact on your health, energy level and how much you enjoy your new eating lifestyle.

Chapter 13: WORKING OUT LESS TO LOOK BETTER THAN EVER

Getting regular exercise, through both cardio exercise and resistance/strength training, is an integral part of losing belly fat. It burns calories, speeds up your metabolism, helps your body to use glucose and regulate insulin and reshapes your body.

The workout program included in the Belly Fat Diet is customizable to you and your preferences, can be done by anyone at any level of fitness, requires only a few pieces of optional, inexpensive equipment and can be done in thirty minutes per day.

Interval Training Basics

As you read earlier, interval training is simply the alternating of moderate work with more intense work. You can use interval training for virtually any cardio exercise, including walking, running, swimming, biking or dancing. With walking and running you can increase the intensity by changing the terrain or increasing speed. With swimming, you can do the crawl for your moderate periods and the butterfly for your intense periods or simply increase your speed. You get the idea.

Interval training is also easily incorporated into strength training or resistance training. You simply alternate a strength training move, such as three sets of biceps curls, with one minute of running on the treadmill, jumping rope or jumping jacks. Any cardio exercise will do, even dancing to your favorite fast song.

Here are some guidelines to keep in mind about interval training:

1. *Always warm up for two minutes, whether you're doing cardio or strength training.*

2. *Always cool down for two minutes by stretching.*

3. *Always begin and end with a moderately paced segment.*

4. *Moderately paced segments should be longer than your intense segments.*

You can adjust the length of each period to suit your fitness level, but it should still remain about 2:1. In other words, the moderate segment should be twice as long as the intense segment. If you walk at a moderate pace for four minutes, you walk uphill or at a faster pace for two, and so on.

Chapter 14: An Overview of the Workout Program

You're going to be able to customize your workouts to meet your needs, likes and fitness level. We provide several options in the next section, but here are the basics.

The goal is to work out for thirty minutes a day, six days a week. You can divide this schedule in a couple of different ways.

Six days a week, you can do the 50/50 Combo Blast, which is fifteen minutes of cardio and fifteen minutes of strength training in one workout. You'd do the same cardio routine each day and alternate the lower body and upper body strength training sessions. That would look something like this:

Monday, Wednesday, Friday: 50/50 Lower Body Combo

Tuesday, Thursday, Saturday: 50/50 Upper Body Combo

Or,

Three days a week you can do one of the cardio workouts and three days a week you can do one of the whole body strength training workouts. So:

Monday, Wednesday, Friday: 30 Minute Cardio Workout

Tuesday, Thursday, Saturday: 30 Minute Strength Training Workout

This workout plan is supposed to be fun, varied and interesting, so feel free to do the 50/50 Workouts for a month and then switch to the 30 Minute Workouts. You can also use walking for your cardio one month and switch to swimming the next. It's best to stick with one plan for a month so that you can properly track your progress and set new goals, but there's nothing wrong with switching it out every month. In fact, it will keep your body guessing and help you avoid that dreaded plateau while you're warding off boredom.

Customizing Your Workouts and Changing Your Workouts as You Progress

Cardio Workouts: We provide several suggested cardio workouts in the next section, but once you feel comfortable with the guidelines, you're free to come up with other ways of getting your cardio. The only caveat is that it be something that you can integrate with interval training easily. Basketball is great exercise, but not necessarily a good candidate for interval training. Rollerblading is, as are rowing, dancing and many other great forms of cardio.

Strength Training: Stick to the suggested routines until you know what you're doing. To make them accessible and affordable to everyone, we've made our routines easy to do at home without expensive equipment. If you want to switch to using a gym later on, or if you already have or want to buy a weight machine or treadmill, you're certainly encouraged to do so.

With cardio, consistency and endurance are more important than speed, so please start off slowly and safely. Interval training allows you to progress more quickly than static training, so you're going to make progress soon enough. If you hurt yourself or become discouraged by starting off at a level that is too difficult for you, you'll sabotage yourself and derail your efforts.

With strength training, maintaining proper form is far more important than the amount of weight you lift or number of reps and sets you do. Again, start off at a level that is appropriate to your fitness level.

Our strength training workouts all use your body weight as resistance. If you like, you can add a resistance band or dumbbell workout later. When you do, you should only lift as much weight as you can lift with perfect form. The last rep should be hard, but if you're in danger of dropping the weight, you're lifting too much.

You're going to see dramatic results from interval training in a very short period of time. Be patient, be safe and have fun.

Chapter 15: AN OVERVIEW OF YOUR MAKEOVER PLAN

Now that you know the components of the Belly Fat Diet, let's put it all together in one easy-to-follow list, so that you can refer to it as needed without having to page through the entire book.

The Eating Plan:

Eat only the foods on the foods list.

Eat as often as possible, with no more than three hours between meals or snacks. Two is better. You can eat three main meals and unlimited snacks or just eat several mini-meals and snacks all day, whichever suits your lifestyle and personality.

Eat as soon after waking as you can, even if it's just a snack.

Eat one sweet treat per day. You can skip it if you don't care for sweets, but you can't have more than one per day.

Once a week, you'll have a planned cheat, according to the guidelines. Take the recommended supplements twice per day, every day.

The Workout Plan:

Target working out for 30 minutes, six days a week, using either the 50/50 Combo Workouts or alternating the 30 Minute Workouts.

Also:

Try to sleep at least seven hours per night at roughly the same time each night, ideally going to bed within the same two hour time period every night.

You want to drink a minimum of 64 ounces of water per day.

Putting the Belly Fat Diet Into Action

- *Two Examples for Your Meal Plans*
- *Tips for Planning Your Meals*
- *Introduction to the Workout Plans*
- *The 50/50 Workout Plans*
- *The 30 Minute Workout Plans*

Chapter 16: TWO EXAMPLES FOR YOUR MEAL PLANS

The Belly Fat Diet Plan is supposed to allow you some freedom of choice in your diet, as well as a simple to follow plan. How you divide your meals is up to your preferences, your lifestyle and your schedule. If you want to graze all day, without planning regular, larger meals, you can do that. If you want to plan three regular meals with several snacks in between, you can do that, too.

Here are a couple of examples that can help you map out the meal plan that works best for you.

A Grazing Plan

(The times are just examples we're using instead of meals)

8am: Dr. Oz's Smoothie or the Sunshine Smoothie

10am: An apple and a cheese stick

12pm: Boiled egg, spinach and tomato wrap with vinaigrette

2pm: Greek yogurt and red grapes

4pm: Coffee, celery sticks with almond butter 6pm: Chicken breast and brown rice soup 8pm: Dark chocolate and an orange

10pm: Green tea and cottage cheese with fresh peaches

A Traditional Meal Plan:

Breakfast:

Scrambled eggs with mushrooms, peppers and onion Slice of whole grain toast with almond butter

Sliced apple Coffee

Morning Snack:

Cheese stick and an orange

Late Morning Snack:

Grapes and almonds

Lunch:

Chicken soup Boiled egg Pineapple spears

Afternoon Snack:

Sesame butter and honey on a slice of whole-grain bread

Dinner:

Broiled salmon

Sautéed spinach, shallots and mushrooms Baked sweet potato

Salad with romaine, red peppers, onion and honey-lime dressing

Evening Snack:

Two slices of watermelon

Late Night Snack:

Greek yogurt

As you can see, you can divide up your food any way you like, plan as much or as little as you prefer and eat as often as you want. Feel free to mix and match days as well, to suit a changing schedule or just to keep things interesting.

The only things you need to do are stick to the foods list and the guidelines.

Chapter 17: TIPS FOR PLANNING YOUR MEALS

Planning meals on a diet can be a real chore. If you try the following tips, however, you might find it's easier than you think!

If you have limited time to cook, you can double the time you do have by doubling the recipe. Instead of roasting one chicken, roast two. Serve one tonight and use the other for sandwiches, salads and soups throughout the week. Instead of baking two sweet potatoes for your dinner, bake four and take the leftovers to work for a quick snack. Instead of making six cups of soup, make twelve and freeze the extra in small containers.

Each weekend, put together a stash of quick snacks for the office. Load up a lunch bag or tote with your favorite fruits, nuts, cheese sticks, yogurts and containers of soup and other standbys and stick it in the fridge until Monday morning. This way, you always have snacks handy and can stick to your diet even when you forget your lunch. It takes a lot less time than packing snacks each morning, too.

Keep an inexpensive blender at work, as well as your favorite protein powder, a small container of milk or almond milk, and a few Ziploc bags of frozen fruit. You'll be able to grab a smoothie when hunger hits or you don't have time for lunch.

Try a few new foods each week. They can either be exotic fruits you've never tasted, types of fish you never knew heard of or just foods you rarely remember to buy. Varying your diet not only keeps it interesting, it also ensures a wide variety of nutrients.

Anticipate cooking challenges. Dieting when you have a family or spouse who isn't joining you can present a tough test of your diet commitment. Don't worry! Many delicious meals can be adapted to the Belly Fat Diet Diet without your loved ones noticing. You can also modify your portion of a meal so that it meets the guidelines. For instance, if you're making barbecued chicken breasts for the kids, just roast yours without sauce. If your husband is having pork chops, sweet potatoes, green beans and a salad, skip the chops, load up on the veggies and heat up a slice of turkey for your plate.

The point is to avoid cooking two separate meals: one for you and one for everyone else. It saves time and energy better spent elsewhere and can also avoid making you feel frustrated and isolated.

INTRODUCTION TO THE WORKOUT PLANS

A Note for Beginners

These workouts are designed so that anyone can do them, without any equipment other than a good pair of shoes. However, if you are completely new to working out and need instruction for specific stretches and the weight training moves, there are plenty of books and DVDs that can help. Better yet, get free help on the internet. Sparkpeople.com, Shape.com and FitnessMagazine.com are all excellent resources for free slide shows and short instruction videos of each move.

Kicking it Up

As you gain strength and endurance, you'll want to kick things up a bit. Do this at your pace and forget about what your friend, spouse or co-worker is doing. Your plan is about you.

To increase the intensity of your cardio workouts, you can simply shorten your moderate segments and lengthen your intense segments, add rougher terrain or even add small dumbbells to a walking workout.

To increase the intensity of your weight training, you can do more reps in the same time, add a resistance band or dumbbells or start using a weight machine. Again, you can find plenty of free videos online that will show you how to do this.

THE 50/50 WORKOUT PLANS

The 50/50 Workout Plans incorporate both cardio and strength training into a 30 minute workout. You'll do the same cardio workout each day, six days a week, choosing from the walking, running, biking or swimming plans.

You'll do the lower body strength training routine and the upper body strength training routine on alternate days. (Both of these include some abdominal exercises, since you can safely and effectively work your abs without a day of rest in between sessions.) Your cardio workouts take 20 minutes and your strength training takes 10.

When you're doing the 50/50 Workout Plans, it's best to start with your cardio. Your resistance training workout goal is muscle fatigue. That's what builds lean muscle fast, but it isn't a good idea to exhaust your muscles right before you head out for a run.

If you're doing your cardio outdoors and strength training at home, don't worry about the downtime in between. Contrary to traditional thought, you don't need do thirty minutes of uninterrupted exercise to reap the benefits; you just need to do the thirty minutes. Of course, if you're raring to go, you can choose an indoor cardio workout so that you can move right on to the strength training.

Cardio

Cardio Workout for Walking Outdoors

2 Minutes: Stretching and warm up — be sure to stretch your neck, shoulders, arms, back and legs.

4 Minutes: Walk at a moderate pace.

2 Minutes: Walk at a fast pace, fast enough to prevent easy conversation. 4 Minutes: Walk at a moderate pace.

2 Minutes: Walk at a fast pace.

4 Minutes: Walk at a moderate pace.

2 Minutes: Cool down by repeating your stretching exercises.

Cardio Workout for Walking or Running on a Treadmill

2 Minutes: Stretching and warm up.

4 Minutes: Walk/run at a moderate pace or on a flat terrain.

2 Minutes: Walk/run at a fast pace or on an incline

4 Minutes: Walk/run at a moderate pace or flat terrain.

2 Minutes: Walk/run at a fast pace or on an incline.

4 Minutes: Walk/run at a moderate pace or on a flat terrain.

2 Minutes: Cool down by repeating your stretching exercises.

Cardio Workout for Running Outdoors

(Recommended only for those already accustomed to running regularly)

2 Minutes: Stretching and warm up.

4 Minutes: Run at a moderate pace on a flat terrain.

2 Minutes: Run sprints or up and down stairs.

4 Minutes: Run at a moderate pace.

2 Minutes: Run sprints or up and down stairs.

4 Minutes: Run at a moderate pace.

2 Minutes: Cool down by repeating stretching exercises.

Cardio Workout for Cycling (Indoors or Outdoors)

2 Minutes: Stretching and warm up.

4 Minutes: Cycle at a moderate pace or low resistance.

2 Minutes: Cycle at a fast pace or higher resistance.

4 Minutes: Cycle at a moderate pace or low resistance.

2 Minutes: Cycle at a fast pace or higher resistance.

4 Minutes: Cycle at a moderate pace or low resistance.

2 Minutes: Cool down by repeating stretching exercises.

Cardio Workout for Swimming

2 Minutes: Stretching and warm up (in or out of the water).

4 Minutes: Swim at a moderate pace using the crawl stroke.

2 Minutes: Swim at a faster pace or using the butterfly stroke.

4 Minutes: Swim at a moderate pace using the crawl stroke.

2 Minutes: Swim at a faster pace or using the butterfly stroke.

4 Minutes: Swim at a moderate pace using the crawl stroke.

2 Minutes: Cool down by repeating stretching exercises.

Lower Body Strength Training Routine

1 Minute: Warm up by stretching.

Do twenty front lunges, five for each leg.

1 Minute: Run in place, jump rope or do jumping jacks. Do ten squats.

1 Minute: Run in place, jump rope, or do jumping jacks. Do twenty hamstring lifts (aka toe raises).

1 Minute: Run in place, jump rope or do jumping jacks. Do twenty leg lifts or reverse crunches.

1 Minute: Run in place, jump rope or do jumping jacks.

Do twenty modified crunches. (Lifting only until shoulders leave the floor.) 1 Minute: Cool down by repeating stretching exercises.

Upper Body Strength Training Routine

1 Minute: Warm up by stretching.

Do twenty pushups. If full body pushups are too difficult, start on your knees with ankles crossed.

1 Minute: Same cardio as above. Do twenty seated chair dips.

1 Minute: Same cardio as above.

Do twenty alternating crunches (aka oblique or scissor crunches). 1 Minute: Same cardio as above.

1 Minute: Cool down by repeating stretching exercises.

THE 30 MINUTE WORKOUT PLANS

The 30 Minute Workout Plans use the same moves and steps as the 50/50 Plans. You're simply combining workouts and doing them on alternating days. Three days per week, say Mon-Wed-Fri, you'll do your cardio workout. The other three days, Tues/Thurs/Sat, you'll do a combined strength training workout. Feel free to switch these days around, they're just an example.

The 30 Minute Cardio Workout

To do the 30 Minute Cardio Workout, simply choose your preferred method of cardio from the 50/50 Plans and double the number of segments, with the exception of the warm up and cool down times.

The 30 Minute Strength Training Workout

2 Minutes: Warm up by stretching.

Do twenty front lunges, five for each leg.

1 Minute: Run in place, jump rope or do jumping jacks. Do ten squats.

1 Minute: Same cardio as above.

Do twenty hamstring lifts (aka toe raises). 1 Minute: Same cardio as above.

Do twenty leg lifts or reverse crunches. 1 Minute: Same cardio as above.

Do twenty modified crunches. (Lifting only until shoulders leave the floor.) 1 Minute: Same cardio as above.

Do twenty alternating crunches (aka oblique or scissor crunches). 1 Minute: Same cardio as above.

Do twenty pushups. If full body pushups are too difficult, start on your knees with ankles crossed.

1 Minute: Same cardio as above.

Do twenty seated chair dips.

1 Minute: Same cardio as above.

2 Minutes: Cool down by repeating stretching exercises.

The Belly Fat Diet Shopping Guide

Vegetables

Alfalfa sprouts

Arugula

Bamboo shoots

Bean sprouts

Beet greens

Beets

Bell peppers

Bok choy

Broccoli

Broccoflower

Brussels sprouts

Cabbage

Carrots

Cauliflower

Chard (Swiss & red)

Chinese cabbage Chives

Collard greens

Garlic

Green onions

Green peas Greens

Horseradish

Kale

Leeks

Lettuce (preferably dark, leafy varieties)

Lima beans

Mushrooms

Mustard greens

Onions

Parsley

Peppers, preferably orange or red Pumpkin

Sauerkraut

Shallot Snow peas

Soy beans

Spinach

Summer squash

Sweet potato & yam

Tomato

Turnip greens

Watercress

Water chestnuts

Winter squash

Fruits

Acai berry — also called the Acai fruit

Apples

Apricot

Avocado

Banana

Blackberries

Black raspberries

Blueberries

Boysenberries

Cantaloupe

Cherries

Clementines

Coconut

Dates Figs Grapefruit Grapes Guava

Honeydew melon

Honey pomelo

Jujube — a subtropical fruit

Lemon Lime

Lingonberries

Mango

Nectarines

Oranges

Papaya

Peaches

Pears

Persimmon

Pineapple

Pitaya or Dragon fruit

Plums

Pomegranate

Raspberries

Star fruit

Strawberries

Tangerines

Ugli fruit

Watermelon

Fish and Seafood

Oily Fish Varieties

Salmon Trout Mackerel

Herring, fresh

Sardines, in water or olive oil

Pilchards

Kipper Eel

Whitebait

Tuna (fresh is best but packed in water is okay, too)

Anchovies

Swordfish

Bloater

Cacha Carp

Hilsa Jack fish

Katla

Orange roughy

Pangas

Sprats

Other Great Fish

Cod

Haddock

Sole

Flounder

Snapper

Catfish

Skate

Whiting Smelt

Shellfish, Mollusks and Misc.

Shrimp Crab

Lobster

Crawfish

Clams

Oysters

Scallops

Prawns

Octopus Squid

Meats and Poultry

Lean beef steaks and roasts, trimmed of all visible fat (limit of one serving per week)

Chicken breast, skin removed

Ground chicken breast meat

Turkey breast, skin removed

Ground turkey breast meat

Eggs

Dairy Products

Skim, 1% or 2% milk

Almond milk

Low-fat or nonfat cottage cheese

Low-fat or part-skim

Mozzarella

Greek Yogurt, probiotic if available

Grains

Brown rice

Whole grain oats

Whole grain hot and cold cereals, no sugar added

Barley

Quinoa

Whole grain bread

Whole grain, whole wheat flour

Whole grain wrap or tortilla

Nuts, Seeds and Oils

Canola oil

Olive oil

Almonds

Brazil nuts

Pecans

Pine nuts

Poppy seeds

Pumpkin seeds

Sesame seeds

Walnuts

Almond butter

Sesame butter

Other Allowed Foods

Balsamic vinegar

Rice vinegar

Mustard

Horseradish

Hot sauce

Soy sauce

Teriyaki sauce

Herbs and Curry

Nori (Seaweed paper)

Whey or Soy protein powder, no sugar

Flax seed

Psyllium husk

Bran flakes

Brown or white sugar

Honey

Agave nectar

Dried blueberries

Dried cranberries

Dried cherries

Dried apricots

Dried peaches

Dried pineapple

Dried figs

Green tea

Black tea

Coffee

Water (lots!)

Sweet Treats

Frozen fruit pops, no sugar Sorbet, no sugar

Dark chocolate, min. 66% cacao

Nonfat pudding

The Shopping Guide

You can use this guide to help plan your grocery shopping or take it with you to use as a section-by-section guide.

For the most part, shopping for the Belly Fat Diet is pretty straightforward: shop around the edges of the store, where the produce, meat, seafood and dairy sections are usually situated. There isn't a whole lot for you in the middle, where the grocery items, convenience foods and snacks are located. We'll cover those areas, too, but you'll be shopping mostly from the perimeter of the store.

The Produce Section

This is one of only two departments where you have almost free reign; the other is the seafood counter. However, there are some things to keep in mind when choosing your produce.

Buy organic as much as you can afford to. If you're on a tight budget, buy organic fruits and veggies if you'll be eating them raw with peel intact, but you can buy traditional varieties if you'll be peeling or cooking them before you eat.

Try to get a wide variety of the power produce items. These are greens that are dark and leafy and fruits, berries and veggies that are dark red, orange or yellow. They have the highest antioxidant and phytonutrient content.

Remember, no white potatoes or corn.

The Seafood Section

When buying fish, opt for the oily varieties first to get that rich Omega-3 content.

When choosing any fish, shellfish and mollusks, fresh is best, even if you'll be freezing it. Make sure it hasn't been thawed from frozen. If it has, you'll need to eat it right away or cook it before you can safely freeze it again.

Fish from the frozen food section is okay to buy, as long as it contains no breading, coatings or sauces.

The Meat Section

Here again, buy organic, grass-fed meats and poultry if at all possible. You'll avoid the hormones, additives and other things your body doesn't need. Kosher products are also a good way to go.

You can buy chicken and turkey breasts with the skin and ribs removed or save a good deal of money by removing them yourself. It isn't hard and only takes a few minutes. You can even use the skins and ribs for making your own stock.

When buying ground chicken or turkey, be sure the label says ground breast meat, not just ground chicken or turkey. Regular ground chicken and turkey often includes dark meat and skin and contain the same amount of fat as a juicy steak.

On the subject of beef, you're looking for leaner cuts of steak and roasts.

Rounds and loins are some of the leaner cuts to consider.

The Dairy Section

Shopping here is pretty simple, since your choices are fairly limited to milk, almond milk, eggs (free range, organic and vegetarian), Greek yogurt (probiotic if available), mozzarella and cottage cheese, both in low or nonfat varieties. You can also find your nonfat pudding here, any flavor you like.

The Frozen Food Section

We've already mentioned that frozen seafood is okay to purchase.

You may also want to pick up frozen veggies without butter or sauce added and frozen fruits without syrup or added sugar.

Other foods you'll find here are frozen fruit bars (the kind with whole fruit, water and nothing else) and sorbet with no added sugar.

The Grocery or Middle Sections

There isn't much here for you, but you'll be picking up a few things. The less time you spend in the center of the store, the less time you'll have to be tempted by cookies, chips and other nasty tidbits. Those are for cheat days and you shouldn't buy them until cheat day. Having them in the house all week is a bad idea.

When buying sandwich bread, wraps or tortillas, make sure they're whole- grain. Whole wheat does not mean whole-grain, so read the labels carefully. Also, you want at least 6 grams of fiber in a slice of bread or it just isn't worth it. Make sure to check for high fructose corn syrup in the ingredients and put the bread back if it's there.

You'll want to pick up brown rice, quinoa, whole grain, steel cut oats and whole, multigrain hot and cold cereals in those aisles.

You can also pick up dried figs, dates, cherries, berries and other fruits here.

Choose those without added sugar.

Other than the allowed condiments, oils, sugar, honey, tea, coffee, spices and herbs, there isn't much else for you here.

CPSIA information can be obtained
at www.ICGtesting.com
Printed in the USA
LVHW011032150521
687531LV00015B/1080